POEMS FOR
Mental & Spiritual Healing

Rufus Johnson

Poems For Mental And Spiritual Healing
Copyright © 2025 by Rufus Johnson

ISBN: 979-8999023025 (hc)
ISBN: 979-8999023001 (sc)
ISBN: 979-8999023018 (e)

Library of Congress Control Number: 2025911881

Rufus Johnson

jrufus52@gmail.com
(804)301-9627

Table of Contents

Acceptance

4-27-2012

Conform to God's will.
His divine will.
Shout with joy for His presence.

Try to walk right.
Only one life to live.
That will be accepted.

Meditate on His goodness
By being righteous
And fearing His power.

Some do not
Stay away from the bad.
The bad will not be accepted.

Our hearts grow closer.
His words get stronger.
We see Him more clearly.

We accept all His grace.
Deliver to us in abundance.
Only real power man has

Is God's power.
Seeking His counsel for guidance.
Our experiences in life

Leads to God.
Our only stable
Reality is with God.

Mold ourselves to His will.
God the Great, I Am.
Looking from above, He sees all.

Observing our hearts
One by one
Through our souls.
Acceptance only counted by our deeds.

America

We love you, America.
You are great, maybe the greatest.
Beautiful like no other.

With gracious skies
From sea to shining sea.
We are trying

To see true America
When all else fails.
We are still here.

And they do drop in.
Granted perfect, you are not.
We all witness.

Need not say or cry.
You are still
Beautiful and we love you.

How can we love another?
When all we have
Is America.

We travel the world.
We are always
Thinking of you.

Housekeeper of the world
Invited and uninvited
All are welcome and they prosper.

We are in pain, America.
Our pain shows through
To keep our freedom.

All that beauty by yourself.
Others wanting what you have.
Wanting to be like you.

How can you copy beauty?
There can only be one America.
Your design of colors.

White for Caucasoid.
Red for the blood that has been shed.
Blue for the sadness of others.

There's never enough
Freedom for all.
They are here.

For your freedom, America.
That we share so freely.
We welcome them all and they stay.

Conflicts of the world
Have started to
Cover your beauty.

They come from across
The seas and borders
For your freedom.

America, will you
Love us the most.
We are here.

Looking for your love.
We give up blood for you.
Will you be ours?

It was not easy at first.
We are still here.
And you are still.

Beautiful America.

Angels around Us

9-28-2005

Angels around us.
Our divine messenger.
Escorting our path.

Treasuring their protection.
Our informal, heavenly existence.
Angels observing our every move.

Not interfering.
Keeping count of what we do.
Every new life

Brings forth an angel of life.
They are sentence
To a revolving life.

Observing their assignment.
A true witness
To our account.

Having all dates and time.
Recorded in the book of time.
It's all signed.

Sealed and handed over.
We cannot speak
Our tongue none void.

Our angel has witnessed.

Anger and Time

9-2-2013

Anger deeply planted.
Grows into hate.
The more you feed anger.

Deeper the roots grow.
Anger will stay.
Heated with a temper.

A heated body of anger.
Waiting for someone
To walk by.

Swimming in anger.
Drowning in misery.
Living with hate.

Because you cannot
Let go of anger
And past experiences.

Only time can heal.
Our angers with time
Grows stronger.

If there's no release
You will feel the pain
In your chest.

Anger has no pity.
It can do a lot of damage.
Damage that cannot be taken away.

Damages that have been done
In your younger years
You still live with.

Time will not heal that.

Between Us

8-2-2012

A blood connection
Between us
That will not separate us.

We together shall not part.
Between us, there's space
Our lives have.

A life connection.
We all age with years.
When time has.

Grown us apart.
Compared opinion.
We are difference.

Our style of living, different.
Different ways of thinking
Distinguishes us.

Between us, Stop signs
And Go signs
Are in place.

Confident we move on.
Pains and hurts
Filled with laughter.

Broken hearts, sorrows of happiness
Goes with the bad times
Between us.

We should keep one another.
Between us, God.
There are we.

Birds

7-05-2007

Clouds, sky, wind breeze.
The sky, a reflection of blue.
The sky with clouds in between.

Birds belong to the sky.
Gracefully they fly.
Landing on a line with perfect balance.

Content in flight.
Wanting a tree for cover.
They do not sing in flight.

They also sleep at night.
Wake up to sunlight
In the morning.

They sing their song.

Cash to the Flow

9-30-2011

No cash, no flow.
That's no way to go.
Flash that cash.

You will get splash for that cash.
Hold up, hands up.
Depart from that cash.

Gone in a flash.
You have nothing to show.
Make some more cash.

To go with the flow.
Pay bills, go places you know.
Need some cash to show.

Business slow, work no show.
People on the go.
Need gas, cannot pay.

You are broke with no cash.
Work all week.
Still no cash to show.

No pay, no place to go.
Government shut down.
No cash.

We all broke with nothing to show.
Everything we do for that cash.
Not just for show.

Survival of the unfit.
Hanging on for life.
One more day.

No time to play.
Get that cash.
To go with the flow.

No cash, no flow, no way.

Change

7-20-2005

Change, no stay the same.
Nothing stays the same.
That's why everything changes.

Change with every passing fashion.
You will not get far.
We cannot change with each day.

From birth to fully grown.
We have changed a lot.
We live for change.

Time move forward
To the future.
Leaving today behind.

Change someone else's life
Try to change yourself first.
Make a difference in someone's life.

When the day turns into night.
Stars come out.
The moonlight glows.

Changes taking place.
Chances are change
Will happen to you.

You cannot stop change
When change starts to move.
This world changing in every way.

We are changing too.
We can truly see.
That miracles are taking place every day.

Choices

9-10-2012

Making decisions determines.
Our future and who we are.
Make the right choice.

Everything a choice.
Every choice that we make counts.
Choices are made every day.

Any choice can be.
A life-changing event.
And may not be the right choice.

You cannot change.
The choices you made.
Once carried out.

Opportunity lose by.
Making wrong decisions.
So many choices to make.

Making decisions never stops.
Options all around, make a stand.
Make a choice, no one can choose for you.

Decisions of a life-changing future.
We have to make difficult decisions in life.
Our choices have been made.

Choices by the blink of an eye.
If you hesitate, it's too late.
Contemplating a decision.

Be quick, time wasting.
Time just ran out.

Compassion

4-19-2012

Compassion for this life.
That will carry us
Through this life.

From day to day.
If there were compassion for this life.
There would not be so must destruction.

Compassion for one another.
That's where we start.
Help the helpless, with the sick.

Some people have no compassion.
For anyone.
No compassion for this life.

Makes a cold heart.
Every day your heart grows.
Just colder than the last.

The day comes.
When you need help.
Need someone.

To show you compassion.
Someone to care for you.
That you are here today.

Bring forth compassion.
That chooses life.
Have a tear for someone.

For God, family, friends.
Protect your compassion.
Let no one steal your compassion from you.

Let not life turn.
Your compassion into hate.
Let not what others do.

Control your compassion.
Compassion comes from the heart.
Let not your mind be troubled.

For lack of compassion.
Your mind should not be
Cold like ice.

Defeat

6-19-2012

We can get past defeat.
By not giving up.
Lose one day, win the next.

Win far more than we lose.
No one wins all the time.
No one wins in everything.

Maybe you have to lose sometimes.
In order to accept defeat.
To win.

Defeated by being scared to fight.
For God, family, and liberty.
For your soul spirit.

Defeated by doing wrong.
Being forced
To do right.

Every day we awake from sleep.
We have defeated yesterday.
So we have a chance.

Not to accept defeats of yesterday.
Light will overcome darkness.
And we can rejoice and live victoriously.

So in the fight of our life.
We find strength to go forward.
Because yesterday, not today.

So in all our life.
We try to do what's right
To live by the light.

We cannot be
Defeated by darkness.

Dominate

4-28-2012

Man was created in God's image.
So was women.
Males and females together.

We were formed through evolution in time.
God was in the evolution business.
Even before Adam and Eve.

Intelligent why we grow.
Intelligent enough to know.
There's something higher than himself.

In the beginning, God
Let evolution take its form
Before He stepped in.

We were believing in all types of objects.
Looking for Him.
That Higher Power.

So God stepped into evolution of man in time.
To claim all that's His.
Even before His chosen people.

He was busy working His plans.
Man dominate the animals of earth.
Man tries to dominate earth.

Our earth just sits.
And rotations.
So we drill into her at will.

The most beautiful of the planet.
Taking care of us.
Every day and night.

Year in and year out.
All we do is destroy her.
Well our, earth tired of us.

Of our complete disrespect.
Of the air and ground.
We drill into her center core.

Looking, wanting, and taking
Her nutrients.
The nutrients we take.

That's our life source.
The wealthier changing now.
Only because of our greed.

The greed to dominate
The earth.

Dreams

8-31-12

Go to sleep on a thought.
It will go away.
Some will be lost.

To illusions of the minds.
A true dream must be.
A focus thought, not a dream.

That means "work."
Daydreaming will not
Make dreams come true.

Work a dream every day.
To live the dream
Before the dream.

You are the dream.
Be true to a dream.
Go to school, "study."

Work that dream every day.
Then your dream.
Not an illusion.

You are not dreaming, "wondering."
Because your dream is real.
You are not asleep.

Your aspirations are "visions"
That came true
Because you aim.

At your dreams.
And made yours come true.
All by the grace of God.

Empty Love

9-27-2012

Searching and not finding.
Looking, hoping to find love.
Pay attention to love.

Inner voice talking to you.
Telling you.
True love, not empty.

When you look for love.
You will not find love.
Your heart full of no love.

Love yourself first.
Then you find love within.
Promise love to grow old with.

Many times you
Missed the mark
To find love.

All in the wrong places.
Empty love
Cannot fulfill your needs.

You merge your heart
With empty feeling.
Empty love cannot.

Be companion for love.
You have traveled
Great distances.

Looking for love.
Your eyes are full with tears.
Frozen in time.

Coldness of your heart.
Too still for love.
There's some comfort in shared love.

Enough

8-6-2005

What you've been through
What I've been through.
Working to no ends.

Useless ends.
Just to start over again.
Trying to make it all.

Trying to catch the wind.
Religion against religion.
People against people.

Enough of that.
Drugs on the increase.
Already enough.

Enough justice with injustice.
Enough inmates fill.
Our jail cells.

Enough stray bullets
Have struck
Innocent victims.

Child abuse on the increase.
Not enough care for our children.
That's enough.

Enough knowledge
Will not determine our future.
Finally having enough.

More than making due.
More than my share.
Enough time together.

Just to be close to you.
Enough strength to carry on.
Enough hope to give, to share.

When today turns into tomorrow.
Enough days
Has already passed.

When we see
The new day sky blue.
We know that

We are truly blessed
For all the days we lasted.

Escape from Negativity

8-30-2005

Escape from negativity.
It appears suddenly over time.
Not aware of its present.

So you are taken by surprise.
It grows like a tree.
With branches and leaves.

Appears from the ones
You love most.
Appears from within yourself.

Many thoughts
Have crossed, your mind.
How can you keep away?

Only you can
Let certain thoughts through.
Your mind.

It has no face, no form, nor voice.
Yet it appears
From all angels.

Negativity, a way of life.
Live a life of positive thinking.
With positive thoughts.

Reject negativity at its core.
To escape its force.
With positive concentration.

A force we most keep.
To fight the battle.
A war of thoughts.

That has overtaken so many.
The battle constantly on.
The word must get out.

That a war is going on.
We are fighting a war
We know nothing about.

Defeated before our time
Because we cannot
Escape from negativity.

Exempt

8-17-2012

Exempt from your responsibilities.
Not being here
In reality.

No one is exempted from responsibilities
Or from rest nor sleep
That our bodies need for life.

We must pay to live.
Nothing for free.
That we must work to live.

We are not set free.
To do at will.
We are subjected to laws.

We should take full
Responsibility for all actions.
No exemption from cause and effect.

A wild life
Leaves missing pieces.
No exemption from self.

Our freedom has a price.
We fight for what's right.
Peace has no immunity.

The freedom that we have.
Are not exempt from bondage.
We are not exempt from our sins.

No one subject to no rules.
The life we lived.
Cannot be exempted from the past.

Fallen Star

9-8-2012

Heavenly elements in the sky.
Falling through space.
Gleaming with subdued light.

Faraway star, coming closer.
Flash of light.
Shooting across the sky.

A sight we long to see.
Then it's gone.
Descending through space.

Extraordinary distances.
They are, seems closer.
Extended traces of light.

The beginning, too far.
The end, too far.
Sparkling through space.

Stars have, their place
In the heavens.
The farthest point.

No one knows.
Stars are eternity.
Some do fall.

Showering their light.
They fill the galaxy.
Suspended in space.

And if one does fall.
We hope it burns out
Before ground.

Forever

12-10-2005

Forever, a moment away.
Forever an hour, who can say?
Forever and a day.

Who can see tomorrow?
Forever, many years away.
Forever, only time can say.

Forever, time never part.
From beginning to end.
Our clock ticking.

Live life cautiously.
For forever only
A moment away.

We move on.
It's here to stay.
We are here to keep forever.

Company for some time.
Warm greeting.
Joyful living.

Welcome a new birth.
Into our forever sphere.
Bound on Mother Earth forever.

Learning, playing, working.
Living in peace together, forever.
Amen.

Forget

9-1-2012

Remember the past
You tried to forget.
Memories kept in mind.

Unintended lack of memory.
Slight of memory, we forget.
Memory lapse, no recall.

Unable to recall past events.
Remember what you want.
Not a bad childhood, treated badly.

You can never forget that
There's much
We need to forget.

Mind tied up
With unwanted, past memories.
Will not be absence from thoughts.

It's hard to forget and forgive.
The truth will not be forgotten.

Freedom

1-17-2003

Freedom to all people.
We live to be free.
To have our freedom.

Without worrying if or not
Can it be taken away?
We fight to be free.

Worried about freedom.
Being threatened
All over the world.

Everyone wants to be free.
To have liberty to speak.
Not to have your voice restrained.

Be able to speak your peace.
Not just saying.
What you want to say.

The truth must be spoken.
Without worrying if.
Your freedom being put in jeopardy.

Without order, there's only chaos.
Limited moral values
Cannot be the standard.

Madness uncovered.
In freedom with no morals values.
Our moral ethics should rule.

What's freedom without rules?
Unorganized chaos
Without rules to govern our conduct.

Our behavior kept under control.
We cannot have freedom without rules.

Give

9-27-2012

The heart, the source of giving.
Without a heart.
The mind will not give.

We need a giving spirit.
Measure giving.
It will never be enough.

Without giving of our hearts.
We cannot bleed happiness.
To give means to sacrifice something.

Because you gave.
Much will be given to you.
Because you gave, no one indebted forever.

Giving should have some pain.
Giving looks for no return.
Give to others.

Give until the heart's content.
It's your right to give.
Be graceful in your giving.

Give more than you receive.
Give freely to all.
Give to the poor, help the needy.

There's a price to pay for giving.
The cost.
Every good deed will be rewarded.

Your return will be low.
Blessing comes by giving.
Cleanse your heart, give.

And what you gave will not add up.

Good

1-17-2013

Good with one o missing
Spells G-o-d.
Try to be good.

With no in between.
There's none.
Can there be one?

For the good we do.
Will not go unrewarded.
And you think.

Why is this so
That this world
We live on is full of sins?

The sins we due.
Controlling our actions.
The sins we make are to ourselves.

We live to do well with others.
And the good you do
Will be rewarded.

Accused of being bad.
When you are good.
There's pressure to be equally balanced.

And your goodness.
Must sustain the bad.
We live between the bad and the good.

We must strive for the good.
Your goodness will suffer.
By the evil that lives.

Lives around and from within.
There's only one cure for the evil
The bad and the ugly.

That's the good Spirit of God
That resides within you.
Every one runs short of goodness.

God, the righteousness one.
Our souls, the messengers
Of our goodness.

Hatred

8-1-2012

Do we love to hate?
Or do we hate to love?
Hating makes some feel better.

Hating makes some smile.
After hurt, they love.
There's no love in hate.

Revenge draws us
Closer to evil.
Drawn into hate.

Obsessed with revenge,
We live with hate.
We start to detest love.

We become hate.
Lovers of weaknesses.
Hungry for more victims.

Evil intensified by our nature.
Arrogance and cruelty, our passions.
Deeply rooted hostilities grow.

Our hatred, full of prejudices.
We haul prejudice around.
From years past events.

That has dragged us down.
Our minds, bodies, and souls
Cannot be filled with hatred.

Our happiness will not
Come from hatred.
Hatred offends life.

We should not live to hate.
Our hearts will not love
Hatred jealousy.

Our souls cannot hate.
Hatred destroys souls.
Our hate has strong ties to evil.

Hatred will not heal.
It only destroys.
We should never savor hate.

Hatred loves its own taste.
It stays in the belly
And has no place to go.

Hatred will win
When the end comes.

Heartbeat

8-15-2005

When your heart beats.
Mine beats too.
What are your thoughts of me?

We were one.
Our thoughts were together.
We thought forever.

A heartbeat away.
From a heartbreak.
Aching hearts skip a beat.

Sorrow follows.
Bring the joy to my mind.
So that I can escape.

From sorrow.
Warm loving.
Heartbeats for me.

We brought ours hearts together.
And you took
My heart and left me.

All I could do was cry.
After the tears were gone.
All that was left was your sting.

Baby, when you left.
A part of me left too.
I feel where you are.

Even when you are not with me.
We are not together.
You still have my heart.

Help Needed

9-14-2012

Assistance, some support needed.
Help always wanted.
Unmeasured help needed.

No ruler can be put on help.
We cannot go through life.
Without some help.

Some people cannot.
Ask for help.
Clearly some help needed.

Some are sentenced on needing help.
Born unable
To take care of self.

In times, of distress.
We all look for some help.
Someone needs to render assistance to you.

To rescue you from poverty.
Relieve you from distress.
Help needed from suffering.

Mentally, you cannot take
Emotional suffering any longer.
Urgent help needed in all conditions.

People need help.
Going through life alone.
Our duty to help one another.

We need to find ways to help.
The helpless.
Sometimes we all need help.

Here

9-21-2012

Tell the world that.
The truth's here.
We must understand.

The truth of why we are here.
The truth must be made clear.
Why we are placed here "for a reason."

The circumstances we face every day.
Prepares us to be here.
Our existence points to the present.

To pave the way.
For the next generation.
Every moment, precious time.

For the children
To become their moment in time.
To prepare for their next generation.

To be here.
Very special, very precious
Moment in time.

Today will be remembered.
We are not permanently placed.
We are a temporary stay.

The picture we paint.
Much bigger than ourselves.
We look into our past.

And wonder why we are here.
It's no accident, us being here.
Our picture has already been painted.

The future, here, now.

Hope

9-15-2012

Downtrodden, depressed in jail.
Misused and abused.
There's always reasons for hope.

Hope has not left home.
There was no peace to see.
It was not to be found.

So hope went its way.
Hope gone for a while.
To look for peace.

Hope, what we live for.
Hope, a feeling
That will not let us go.

Just say I have hope.
Hope has arrived.
Hope has come home.

Come home to the hopeless.
Find strength in hope.
Grounded and anchored in God.

All we can do is hope.
That it never leaves us.
Hope always on top of today.

Looking at tomorrow.
Work for hope, look for hope.
And we will see a better tomorrow.

I Can

8-15-2012

I can tell you.
About my life.
I can tell you some right and wrong.

You must do what's best for yourself.
I cannot know.
The better part of you.

Than you know yourself.
First we are strangers.
Then I can listen to you.

I cannot fight your battles.
Your battles for the Lord.
He fights for you.

I can look to the sky
And see the stars at night.
I can make a difference in this world.

I can start by making.
A difference in myself first.
Then spread the seeds.

Of help around.
That others can see.
The good that help will do.

I can see the trees.
I can feel the wind.
Blow pass the seasons.

And see the birds fly
Through the sky.
I cannot see God.

I do feel that I know
When He is near.
I can feel His presence near.

In the Sands

4-1-2012

My heart, mind, and soul.
Belong to you, Lord God.
My understanding, not enough.

Lord, your words
Give life to me.
Knowledge of you brings wisdom.

I look for you in everything I do.
Your protection, already in place.
Lord God, teach me how to pray.

Teach me how to live.
Live for you today.
My end, I have not seen.

Answering to you.
Preparing myself
For that ultimate test.

Looking at events of my past.
Out of my control.
I see you taking over.

Like never before.
And carrying me
Through it all.

Looking at my footprints
In the sands.
I see you, Lord, in charge.

Holding me in the sands.
Taking care of me.
My distress, in your hands like never before.

Never before have I
Looked into the sands
With meaning.

Never before have I
Looked into the sands
With understanding of your power and might.

Never before have I
Look into the sands
And understood your love for me.

In the sands.

Incomplete Path

11-19-2012

A collection of broken trails.
Recycled memories not in use.
Stacks of unsolved problems.

A polluted mind
With incomplete thoughts.
Time spent going toward a broken trail.

A faraway place.
No one sure of its ending.
Your feet trodden by yesterday's walks.

Each day on
The trail of life.
We move on still farther.

Into incomplete paths.
Moving on in life's path.
Leaving an impression of today's path.

With actions, conducted footsteps.
Incomplete purpose needs directions.
A purpose with directions.

That shows us the right way to go
Toward a completed path.

Jesus Christ

9-10-2012

Jesus the Lamb of God, also the Son of God.
The Messiah, the Life for the World.
Deliverer of compassion.

A teacher of morality.
Trust in His teaching.
He fulfilled God's promise through sacrifice.

Christ's teaching, a reachable goal.
No Christian should be without His teaching.
The New Testament starts with Jesus and the old ends.

The flesh of God came to us.
Be not recognized, the Savior
And His own, received Him not.

We cleave to His memory for salvation.
He was sent by the Father with the sword of wisdom.
We live by His salvation.

Guiding hope, some suffering.
Release sins to Christ.
Sinners do seek recovery.

When brought low
In life
We run to Jesus.

Christ born of a virgin.
Lowly in life, with animals.
Laid in their bed, for His bed.

Crucified, came back to life.
Walked the earth again.
To recover lost souls.

Now next to the Father, there's Jesus.
In the Kingdom with a throne.
He stands victorious over earth.

Knocks

9-15-2012

Knock on the door
Of opportunity.
Someone always knocking.

On that door.
A door that will not open.
A wall with no entrance.

A door with no key.
No entry without permission.
We all, waiting in line.

Knock on the doors of success.
Work your way to the top.
And wait for a door to open.

Knock on the door of heaven.
Find peace within and enter.
No barrier can stop.

You from knocking
On the doors
Of opportunity.

In our journey
Of being knocked around
In life.

We go to the school.
Of hard knocks
From childhood to adulthood.

We learn to knock
On every door before we enter.
Opportunities move in steps.

Keep knocking
On that door at opportunity.
It will open.

Let Me Go

11-21-2005

Let me go.
I want to go.
I cannot take it anymore.

I stayed too long.
I should have been gone.
A long time ago.

And when I am gone.
I want to see.
Smiles for me.

For all the beautiful places.
I will see.
Go while you still have a chance.

To keep from going.
You find reasons to stay.

Life Mountains

8-31-2012

Life Mountains, a far journey.
We walking years just to get started.
How far can we go in life?

Over years and through decades.
No turning back from life's path.
Crossroads of decisions must be made.

Which way will life take us?
Mountains, tribulations and trials.
To get to the other side of life.

Life Mountain, manifested itself
Into life
With understanding.

Life, our compensation.
Our reward, living
After a lifetime of working.

We move forward.
Never giving up.
Stay the course.

Stay focus on Life Mountains.

Life Spirit

10-2-2004

When we were born
A spirit manifested
Itself into life.

We cry into life.
We grow into
Life Spirit every day.

A special existence
Unites us.
Universal harmony connects us.

The power of life
In the veins
Brings forth new life.

For another soul
To live, to reproduce
Our existence in life.

Our life connection.
The Soul.
Descendant at birth, we are kin.

Disharmony within, no connection.
We grow apart.
And we retreat to ourselves.

Life saturations, we made decisions.
Our decisions took.
Us in different directions.

Life report will not lie.
Life lived for the truth.
No lies will be covered.

Our life has spoken.

Love Conquers

8-8-2012

Love grows by the days.
Love has power
Over the lonely heart.

Love prevails over agony.
Nothing exists without love.
A tree will not grow.

Without nature, that's love.
An exquisite flower
Will not grow without care.

Shows that life, lives on love.
A baby before birth
Needs to be loved.

Born by love.
Love must be continued
To see a future.

Our care for this
New life must not stop.
It's just getting started with love.

Our eyes look into their eyes.
We behold a new life.
And cry with tears of joy.

Now we are looking
Into the eyes of love.
Our life for that life, if need be.

To show our love for thee.
Together we
Share the life.

The care you give
Tells the truth about your love.
The love you shared paves the way.

When grown up
You look back through years gone by.
Then you have seen.

Love conquers.

Lying Mirror

11-17-2012

My mirror, only a reflection.
Of what I see.
A reflection of the surface of me.

Reflections cannot see
Past the skin.
My mirror, looking back at me.

The outside will reflect what's within.
The good and the bad
Will show through reflections.

My mirror, telling me
The truth of what I see.
That image shown, that's not me.

My mirror, lying to me.
My mirror, looking back.
On years of reflections.

Looking hard at me.
Still, I cannot see.
All the years gone by.

Where's my refection of yesterday.
My mirror, judging me.
On what I see today.

Mirrors have no sense of time.
This reflection I see, it's real.
Years of truth being told here.

About what I see.
My eyes, looking back
Years of me.

Surely no lies are being told here.
I remember yesterday's years.
This, my reflection today.

And that's no lie.

Make Up

8-25-2005

Make up to break up.
No more.
Yet, I go back for more.

I am hurting.
My heart's broken.
Nerves, shocked up.

My eyes, seeing things.
You will not explain.
Turn then sell out

To the closest bidder.
You must be pitching.
A no-hitter.

I cannot understand
What you say
Nor what you do.

Comparing you seems
To be not one, but two.
What have you not told?

Between us
No one else need know.
Privacy matters, see.

Left alone, will we forget?
Or will we grow closer
The farther we get.

Far away, we cannot stay
Together.
We cannot play.

Tug of war, both pulling
In different directions
With all our might.

And letting go without a fight.
When one quits, no one wins.
Break up no more.

Numbers

Written by
Rufus Johnson Jr.
9-25-2010

No beginning with no end.
Numbers have value.
There has never been a time.

Without numbers
We need some way
To count the years with the days.

Numbers have endured time.
We all classified by numbers.
We the people have strength in numbers.

The total number of people
Changes every second.
Numbers count our population.

A number cannot
Repeat its value.
At the same point in time.

We encounter numbers every day.
We live by
Numbers and a name.

Every computer controlled
By binary numbers.
Computer run the world now.

Imagine if there were no numbers.
We be lost in time.
Blinded by the day and night.

Our hearts must beat
A certain number per minute
For us to live.

Everything measured in numbers.
Numbers set the stage
From beginning to end.

Order

5-20-2005

We love you, God.
Our thoughts are of you.
We wonder about you.

No one knows
Who you really are.
A mystery to us all.

Only your order continues.
Beyond space, there's no end.
You are real.

Our perception of you
A myth.
You are not an illusion.

Your order brings us order.
Those who love you will follow.
Some will not.

Water flows, sun shines.
Evening lights.
Mountains grow.

And we are placed in space.
All set to God's order
With a purpose.

Still, some say that
His presence, not real.
That He, God

Did not create all this.
Creations.
All space, the Milky Way, far galaxies, this universe.

When we were unaware.
Living in caves.
No shelter.

We evolved.
Just to question our Maker.

Our Souls

11-27-2012

The making of us.
Was brought into existence.
By our Maker.

Before the day
We were born
No one can be compared to another.

Our souls transformed earth.
Intelligence gives us dominion
Over the animals.

By the principles of
Our embedded souls.
There's life in our souls.

Our soul makes
Life move for us.
Our soul cries for us to move.

When we grow
Our soul grows with us.
We are one in two.

Is this why the soul grows too?
Our soul requires
Growth for survival.

Circumstances transform into action.
Our soul fighting
Through years of life.

Deep under the skin
We live and grow together.

Out

8-25-2012

Society, out of control.
Respect for authority, nonexistent.
No respect for life.

The lamp low.
Burning with little fuel.
Society, put on notice.

Our existence runs on time.
Time never runs out.
On the other hand.

Our time runs on time
Before the finish line.
Our time has limits.

The most among us
Are limited to a sudden amount of time.
All meets their time out.

Ignorance runs out of time.
Bankrupt for time.
There's only one way out.

A distress call for mercy.
Before time runs out.
To see your way out.

Path

9-27-2012

Endless path.
The path less traveled.
A forgotten path.

Make your own path
On fresh pavement.
No one else has taken

On a path
No one wants to take.
Not the right path.

Put one foot in front of the other.
Each step forward.
Look where you are walking.

Look at your path
Right before your eyes.
Each step, different.

All paths lead
Some place different.
A continue path.

Life path, not straight.
There's always a caution sign.
Always something to look out for.

We have some
Surprising turns
On our pathway through life.

We make wrong choices.
Going no place
In the wrong direction.

We need
To find our
Way home.

Peace Be Still

1-14-2002

Peace be still.
Peace cannot be still.
Our peace needs to move.

From under that rock
She's been hiding for so long.
Hiding from us.

She's afraid.
We stand for you now
Peace.

You do not have to
Hide any longer.
We are here.

To stand by your side.
Peace never arrive.
By fighting, always a loser.

War need not be
For the peace
We seek.

Unruffled anger
Of discontented hate.
Looking for peace through war.

We need to walk with peace.
We need to talk with peace.
We need to believe in peace.

Peace be your defense
From soul to soul.
Then ask peace to be still.

Pray for Healing

8-4-2005

Overexert ourselves.
We will be brought low.
Demanding our dues.

We will get none.
First last, and last first.
God our strength and beginning.

Jesus, please
Hear our prayers
So that we can receive

Your healing power.
Remembering your name.
Our hearts can be healed.

Pray for healing.
Prayer costs nothing.
Time costs, this time not ours.

Then our time, everything.
Our time's been set.
We know not the place.

Our prayers.
We pray for sick and shut-in
Healing.

Pray for those
Who cannot help themselves?
To help one another.

No one fool.
Not being misled
To be paper.

In the wind.
Having defense.
Take cover from the wind.

A believeth we
Can be saved
From the winds.

We must keep ourselves
To see
The true colors of the rainbow.

Pure clouds in the sky
And the wind
Carried masterpieces every day.

Protection

9-15-2012

Defend yourself from harm's way.
Wrongful events can occur.
No safety truly assured.

Have no armor, need some defense.
Avoid violence, if you can.
Guns cannot be our only protection.

We are the enemy.
Protection from ourselves.
Defeated with self-inflicted wounds.

Do not defeat yourselves with self-destruction.
Fight against personal intent.
By understanding, our actions have effect.

Learning produce wisdom.
That's some form of protection.
Every experience we should learn to protect ourselves.

Protection, unprotected sex.
Sex of self-destruction.
We must be conscious of the protection we seek.

Carry ourselves in a way.
For protection to be granted.
Let God be our protector.

Put Down

10-1-2012

Brought low in self-esteem.
Made to feel
Less important.

Making someone to have
No confidence in themselves.

Making someone
Not like their self-worth.
Put someone down.

To pick yourself up.
Being put down.
Not your limitation.

Descending to
A low position.
Not your position.

Channeling
A native state of mind.
Not your mind.

In flame words.
You did not speak them.
People do not define you.

You are not low in status.
Dejected.
Do not lose self-encouragement.

To declare
Your way to self-confidence.
Not to let anyone.

Take you down.
A downward spiral.
Refuse to go to their level.

If you cannot lift
Someone up
Then leave them alone.

Set an example.
Be a builder of confidence.
Raise someone up.

Relax

9-11-2012

Comfort in mind.
Relieve tensions
With milder thoughts.

No need to worry
Over the unchangeable.
Take yourself from commotions.

Feel the effect of quietness.
Do not take any disturbance.
Just close your eyes.

And release all anxieties.
Try not to think.
A stressful mind grows weary.

Not for one day
Will anyone escape reality.
Let go.

Become less stressful.
Release stress.
That's good for mind health.

Better for the nerves.
Problems will continue
Each night.

Let go of today.
Surrender all of today and sleep.
The sun rises on all souls.

Relax, it's a new day.

Remembrance

8-19-2004

Remember the brave-hearted warriors.
Extraordinary once, they were.
Your service completed.

A soldier for us all.
The direction of your life
Was not to be a follower.

So you went your way to serve.
To serve your country.
You did sign for service.

We stand by our signatures in life.
We live by the word we give.
Their word and honor they gave.

Until the end, it showed nonvoid.
Not knowing their return.
To the love ones they left at home.

Your presence will be missed.
We will love you until our end.
We cannot fill your shoes.

Feel your pains.
Know your strengths.
The will to live to the end.

You have fallen among many.
You fought for us.
So that we may live in peace.

Your life will not be forgotten.
To have lived
And fallen in vain.

Cannot be.
Our history filled with the fallen.
Let not there be others.

Our remembrance of you cannot be in vain.

Restless Soul

11-14-2002

Restless soul of me.
We wander where we will be.
Can I control my soul over me?

We are wandering restlessly.
How will my soul feel next?
My soul has emotions too.

Quiet, stop, and meditate.
We start to meet.
Not a clear enough focus.

To understand
So we keep wandering.
Not knowing.

The real purpose of me.
The universe takes us both.
We are not alone.

Others wandering too
For a space.
Life, the only soul that matters.

Our soul wanders over.
Wandering, looking to find our way home.
Not remembering what's happening.

While we are wandering.
From place to place.
Over the same path like others.

Overseas, time and space.
Still looking, hoping
To find reasons.

Why we are wandering?
We are wandering
Because we are looking for peace.

Seasons

10-3-2012

There are reasons for seasons.
Spring into harvest, food will grow.
Colors start to fill the atmosphere.

Summer time hot.
With the sun beaming.
Clouds suspended, we look for shade.

When the leaves fall
To the ground.
It's fall time.

Then we fall back in time.
Getting the ground
Prepared for winter.

A dreary time of the year.
Special days will arrive.
To bring joy for all.

Snowflakes fall
To makes the air cleaner.
The ground purer.

Seasons are determined
By temperature and time of year.
All weather conditions affect the way we dress.

Spring into action.
Be ready and prepared
For all seasons.

Seed

12-15-2005

Fruits of life.
Fruits and flowers
Flourishes in the spring.

Fall, winter's gone, summer's warm.
Smallest seed
Grew the largest tree.

Minerals far below us.
Digging for riches
And destroying our resources.

One day, maybe
No trees grow.
No beauty.

For no flowers grow.
Where did the flowers go?
Busy like a bee.

We are with no time
To plant seeds.
For there is beauty in the seed.

Different seeds for all of us.
What will be said of you?
Seed of a family.

Seeds of giving a helping hand gracefully.
A lovely smile with no content.
A passionate heart.

A mind that will not harm.
No one turns from anger.
Our Lord Jesus turns from anger.

And His blood
Stains our cross.
His seed of compassion

Lives to this very day.
Therefore a seed
Can grow and change this world.

Sleep

11-25-2012

Sleep, a natural
Bodily function.
You are suspended

In sleep, motionless.
A rested body lies dormant
While transcending.

In sleep, we dream.
Resting peacefully.
Our body depends on sleep.

Our body and mind need sleep.
Our heart needs sleep.
All closed eyes are not asleep.

Meditating in mind
We wait for sleep.
In a state of consciousness.

We do not see sleep.
In a state of unconsciousness
We are in sleep.

The exact time, unknown.
We are in a dream.
A world of sleep.

Drifting through sleep.
We wake up, well rested.

So Much to Be Thankful For

6-4-2005

There's so much
To be thankful for.
I cannot keep it to myself.

I cannot tell it all.
Knowing that there's
Nothing out of reach.

I have bowed down and submitted
And I do thank
God for everything.

When my troubles
Start to arise
I pray for faith.

To keep me warm and safe.
To keep my dreams alive.
There is so much for us

To be thankful for.
We should not
Keep it to ourselves.

We must share His bounty.
Tell the world what
He has done for you.

There's no limit set.
On what He can do for us.
Then we all should

Bow down and submit
And we all
Thank God for everything.

There's no limit set on what
He will not do for us.
To keep our dreams alive.

Someone

12-11-2012

Everyone wants and should be
Treated with respect.
Like they are someone.

Make people treat you
Like they want
To be treated.

If you are someone
You should not be
Lowered by any one.

What others say about us
Does not determine our worth.
Our worth should not

Be measured in dollars.
Socially not accepted
You're still someone.

What we think of ourselves
What I think of myself
Makes all the difference.

What others think
Does not make you.
We are more than what people say.

You are better off
To keep trying
To be someone

Than being satisfied
Being called a no one
By someone with lack of funds.

Money does not make you someone.
A fool with money
They will soon part.

Make a decision
To become someone.
With knowledge, you are someone.

Stay

9-17-2014

Stay, never go.
Where will you go to?
If you do not stay.

Away temporarily.
Not wanting to stay.
Away from me, you stay.

Beyond my reach.
I wait for you.
Firmly fixed in my memory.

There you are in my mind.
There you stay.
Some kind of connection we have.

Family may be friend.
Over time, they stay in memory.
The duration of that memory

Should have passed, but they stayed.
Your picture stays in my mind.
Awake, you are still there.

You can go now.
You do not have to stay.
There was a time

When you could have stayed.
You would not.
Yesterday's gone.

Now you can stay gone.

Stop

8-22-2012

To stop a long, enduring habit
That's very difficult to do.
Many have tried in vain.

Some tell you to stop.
You just cannot.
A habit, very troublesome to break.

Reframe from persistence.
Reaching that point to stop.
And you just could not.

Life path, with trials and tribulations.
Make a habit long enduring.
Reflection of the future.

You need to stop.
A halted journey
By a bad habit.

Misguided minds
Move with caution.
Time to stop and reflect.

Everything comes to
A stop eventually.
We all must stop before it's too late.

Strange

8-18-2012

Mystified by unusual events.
Strange things are happening.
Bizarre events taking the world.

And we, the people
Getting stranger every day.
Unexplainable seems normal.

The skies looking strange.
The air changing in a strange way.
Changing times always strange.

We are in changing times.
Unsolved mysteries, happening now.
Strange stories, being told.

The truth needs to be told.
Lies need to move on.
To invest in more lies.

Theirs microwaves of sounds in the air.
Those strange voices.
That so many seem to hear.

Hearing strange sounds.
Never complete silence.
Always that strange ring.

Extraordinary changes taking place.
Then we step into new times.
That seems strange.

Originally alienated, you try to fit in.
Normally you are the strange one.
Today's times you'll fit in.

Nobody's strange, all of us, we are the same.

Street Life

9-25-2012

Life in the fast lane.
You made that choice.
To live the street life.

Your job to work the streets.
Looking for someone to hustle.
Or maybe to get your hustle on.

All hustles in the streets, not illegal.
Some people feed
Their families through street life.

Some live in the streets not by choice.
They do not have a home.
The cold rain, there's no cover.

The streets, that's their home.
They do not love the street life.
That's not their real home.

Grown up, street-smart.
Not smart enough to stay out of jail.
We do need some street smarts.

To get by in today's society.
Thinking you are too street-smart.
You hit that door with no key.

Locked away from your streets.
No way to escape.
Your pavement of

Concrete gold has disappeared.
When you get out
Find yourself a home.

Hold on for a better life.
The street life.
That's no way to live.

Success

9-5-2012

Success is not given; it's earned.
No pain, no gain.
Work hard every day.

Persistence leads to success.
Your goals will not be accomplished
If you ever stop.

To push forward, not to giving up
Before you reach your goals.
Failures only come from stopping too soon.

Preparation, be prepared
For the future.
Strive to achieve prosperity.

To be prosperous in life.
To accomplish and be recognized for your works.
Success must be your intention.

Few manage to maintain full success.
With success comes responsibilities.
Success carries weight and has its victims.

Prepare for the future.
Measure of success.
Money, power, respect, and a balance life.

With God first.

Surrender to Love

6-7-2013

Surrender to love or be alone
And be defeated by love.
You have to feel love.

To understand love
Have passion for love.
Surrender to love for affection.

Embrace your desire to be loved.
Engage time together.
Tender, warm affection for love.

Surrender to love.
Be devoted to love.
Endure years of love.

When love has taken you
To love's end.
Be no fool for love.

You stood by love.
When there was no love
Keep love alive from within.

Love keeps us at peace.
Love loves the truth.
Surrender to the truth.

Love is the truth.
Surrender to love.
Is that the truth?

Thank You

12-7-2012

Thank you, Lord God.
In the morning
When I awake, I give thanks.

My gratitude, shown by antic.
Show your gratitude
By living right by God.

Always remember that
We live by His grace.
Each day has uncontrollable saturations.

We live through them all
And we grow stronger by the day.
Through our faith in You.

Gives us strength
To make each day.
We give thanks to You.

We appreciate You with our deeds
Which speaks for our works.
Our space cannot exist without You.

Our daily journey.
We are subject to You.
Lord, thank you for waiting.

For me, it took some time
For me to arrive
To a place that I know.

That it's You that gets all the praises.
You alone receives all of me.
To You, God, be all the glory.

And to You, we give all thanks.

This World

9-2-2012

This world, a sphere.
Place in space.
And we are earth.

To live for the good.
To love this world
For the beautiful skies.

This world, here for us to live.
To be treated with respect
Like your mother.

We are on Mother Earth
For better or worse.
Like a marriage till we part.

We stand up right, upside down.
Our domain gravitates through ether
That places all matters.

In our world, we live
Our life, set every day.
For our earth, just another day.

Same thing, different day for our earth.
The earth keeps us, not we keep earth.
Everything will grow.

With or without us.
God's the earth keeper and ours.
He keeps all.

Thunder and lightning

8-25-12

Thunder and lightning, a natural force.
We should fear the power
And remove ourselves from its presence.

It strikes with a deadly force.
Illuminates the sky with light.
A combustion of power and might.

Clouds burst
And explosion in the sky
Cutting through the atmosphere.

Lightning the light.
Thunder the explosion of sound.
Nothing reckons the force of lightning.

Strength to command the sky.
To force a violence reaction
In the cloudy atmosphere.

It appears cloudy all day.
Just to release its power
Nothing stands in the way.

The thunder roars, lightning strikes.
Clouds appears darken, no shinning sun.
A loud sound, take shelter.

Lighting coming.

Time

9-19-2012

Life gradually passes time.
Each day consumes
Hours of unnoticed time.

Each day should prove
More productive than the last.
We consume years of time.

That cannot be replaced.
Time, the winner every time.
Years diminished by wasted time.

Well into our years
Our mind grows weary.
Deep, we look into past decades.

At what went wrong.
Long before we knew
Time has passed us by.

Useless time spent.
A sense of a wasted life.
All good times all the time.

One time for all.
We are given in this life.
A priceless gift that we have.

Here, time not to be wasted.
Destructive to the mind, idle time.
No refund on time

Time, a real fact in life.
Time: the past, present, and future.
Time never stops itself.

To Know You

6-7-2013

Been in love with you
Ever since we met.
You started to talk to me.

Consumed by your ways
I could not get away.
Just talking to you

Made me want to stay.
I am interested in you.
To knowing you

So that I can
Care for you.
Seeing you smile

Means the world to me.
Seeing you not smiling
Makes me sad too.

And wondering what to do.
Not knowing what to do.
With growing pains

Added on to years of problems unsolved.
How many more years will it take for us to know.
Sex has nothing to do with love.

What's sex anyway?
Love or no love.
Or do we just want to relieve ourselves.

Love you without sex.
How far will our love go?
Far beyond sex.

A relationship
A friend in need.
A friend indeed.

Blinded by sex for love.
Sex will destroy our love.
That's why getting to know you.

Means so much.
Because sex, not love.

Too Far

4-13-2012

We have come too far
From the beginning.
Too far from the end.

To reach that distant place.
We have come too far
To turn back.

Too far from where we started from.
To where we need to be.
Now that we have come this far.

Seems that we have reached an end.
A road of no return.
We have come too far.

Too far in the wrong direction
To go forward.
Have we come far enough?

To reach our true selves.
Our soul be with us.
Yet far away to hold.

Our souls talk to us.
Walk with us.
God, please be with us.

Do not stay too far away.
Fear from being too far from home.
The planets are too far away.

For man to travel
The universe, too wide.
Too deep to reach an end.

How far can our minds go?
Consciously or unconsciously.
Know that God's not too far away.

Treasure Today

8-8-2012

God brought me through today.
Yesterday and my sorrows.
He brought me through my trials.

Tribulations and pains.
My life I have only through His mercy.
And grace that I live to see.

The light of this day.
Another day the light brought forth.
By His guiding hands.

I am blessed more today
Than I realized yesterday.
More than a blessing to walk.

Through this life, feeling blessed.
Blessing from heaven.
Blessings are God's gift to us.

The gifts of life, finance, and health.
Every day, He gives us food.
Enough food to make another day.

And strength to stay the course.
We are witnessing today.
For tomorrow will be sustained.

Set an example.
Its precious times today.
Our future will tell.

Our stories of yesterday.
That's the lessons for today.
The life that we have lived.

We should treasure today.
Cherish each day we live.
In this moment in time.

This moment in time.
Will not be the same tomorrow.
So treasure today.

Treatment

9-10-2012

People are being mistreated every day.
Treated with disrespect.
Treat others like you want to be treated.

Treat all.
With kindness and respect.
Treat someone you.

Dislike with a distance.
Try to stay away.
Procure your distance.

This treatment makes
People leave their
Home and home country.

People leave jobs
Because of bad treatments.
We want to be treated right.

That will make a difference.
Whether we be friend or foe.
Treatment matters not lightly.

Every one you meet
Becomes treatment to us.
How you treat others.

That's where treatment begins.
At home, from birth.
Treatment in motion.

Somehow treatment
Stays with us.
It will never leave us.

People will treat you
Bad in some form.
Or fashion your whole life.

Somehow we must stay.
Vigorous in our life.
To stay focused.

On our treatment in our life.
To become friends.
We must treat.

One another, equally fair.
This where universal karma steps in.
And it will always

Be in effect
And come back for revenge.

Tricks

10-2-2012

Tricks are being played every day
On the mental of our being.
Nothing what it seems to be.

Believe half of what you see.
Nothing of what you hear.
Spoken words under mind.

Saying something then denied spoken.
Mischievous-worded friends
Deceive with intended wrongs.

A wolf's cries be heard.
The cries go into the air.
No one answers the cries of a wolf.

Tricky love amuses some.
Involving deep feeling
Being played with.

We all fools
That play with love.
Love no toy.

Love an art to some.
Make an art of playing with love.
Who gets tricked in the end?

Uncertainty

9-21-2003

The world full of uncertainty.
Today in time for sure.
Certainty has peace for comfort.

The state of certainty
Brings peace.
Uncertainty exists in every area.

There's no peace
With uncertainty.
There's nothing to be certain of.

No known certainty to show.
No place to go for help.
We accept our circumstances.

Each day more
Unpredictable than the last.
We settle for unsettled happiness.

Saturations has its instances.
Any of our affairs
Could not go our way.

There's always
Something left
For chance.

Nothing definite.
Everything, subject to chance.
Foreseen future cannot be predicted.

Life grows unsettled.
Certainty in survival mode.
Many cries.

To be sure of something
We endure uncertainty.
Still, we prevail.

When we set and wander
And think about
Each day that.

We prevail another day.
With all that happening
In the world.

It's amazing.
With nothing definite
That we make a day.

Count it all being blessed
In a world of confusion.
Complex situations in motion.

Confusion, the word of the day.
For certain, the clock ticking.
And time will win in the end.

Understand

9-14-2012

Understand we are
In evolution.
This the order of life.

Which it operates with perplexity.
Not knowing the real
Purpose of us, we struggle.

Survival knows no bounds.
We walk through life
Without a purpose.

Not knowing
Our next move.
Seize some understanding.

At all time.
It will take time
To comprehend this life.

Understanding accepts changes.
All things will change
At some point in time.

So we change
With the changing time
To understand what

Type of change, taking place.
Understand that if
We do not keep up

We will get left behind.
Understand that we are
In serious times.

So live life seriously.
This life, all we have.
There are consequences

For not understanding
That it's a high price
To pay for ignorance.

Unspoken Words

9-20-2012

Expression with no words.
Broken speech with no action.
Implied action with no words.

A message of a feeling with no words.
That cannot be
Expressed by words.

Action does speak louder than words.
Explosive emotions
Will get us into trouble.

Explosive action without words.
A lot can happen
When we are faced with nothing to say.

Our eyes can speak.
They will tell the whole story
Without saying a word.

Our mouths cannot speak.
Not a word we can say.
To bring comfort to ourselves.

Our voices cannot be heard.
If we speak no one.
Will be spared, tears will flow.

No feeling will be saved.
There will be no peace between us.
Hearts will be shredded.

By what already has been said.
Spoken words cannot be replaced
By unspoken words.
We live by spoken words.

Unthinkable

5-5-2007

When I think of you
Are you thinking of me?
For every second of the day.

My thoughts are of you.
One minute unthinkable.
Because

You carry me through the day.
It is the only way.
All my ways have been futile.

If I thought for one second.
That the glory I see.
And take for myself.

Will not be
Because I cannot
Take glory from thee.

And still seek the Almighty.

Wasting

9-19-2012

Your money has departed.
Useless spending
Has consumed it all.

There's nothing to show
For unproductive spending.
Each dollar should be accounted.

You have failed to be accountable.
Your neglect will be noticed.
Diminish sustain.

No value in your exchange.
Money being wasted.
Everyone will know.

They see the money go
And the years go by.
You achieve nothing.

With your money.
All these years
You have nothing to show.

By overspending, maybe
No one wants to hear excuses
With nothing to show.

It all seems wasted.
Money worthless.
We, you and I

Need to spend more wisely.
Stop overspending
By stop wasting.

There's no value in wasted currency.
Coin, paper, or plastic.
It's all currency being wasted.

What Will Be

7-19-2007

What are you looking for?
To be with your mate.
To stay together.

Not just string along.
Spend time with one another.
To share your life.

Wanting romance.
Not just a one-day stance.
Finally, we are together.

For an explosive moment.
A passionate moment.
We must know the truth

About one another.
The truth may hurt.
One of us, if not both.

Will we stay?
Or
Will we depart and be no more.

Whatever

10-1-2012

Whatever seems to be?
The word of the day?
Whatever happened today?

Forgotten tomorrow maybe.
Any problem can be on alert.
At any given time.

Anything can happen in a day.
Whatever happens, be prepared.
Stay ready for anything.

What you might need in supplies.
Somehow they do to appear.
By some means.

Add all the days
That you have lived.
And you will see that.

All of your whatever.
What you needed.
All has been met.

So God has supplied.
All your needs.

Who Cares

12-14-2012

This day, in time.
No one shows concern.
Yesterday, did we care more?

Suffering and sorrows of the past.
Shows violence and uncaring.
That's the way of the world.

Not to care for anyone.
Who cares for you today?
For a better tomorrow.

Who cares about your problems?
About the injustice
Placed on poor people.

No one cares, it seems.
For someone else's problems.
No one really cares for others.

Will they not sleep?
Because of your problems.
Then who cares?

You start to bleed.
Care about stop bleeding.
Sick, care about getting well.

The world changing.
Does anyone care?

Why Worry

9-17-2012

Feel at ease with no worries.
Release yourself from worries.
Free your thoughts.

Set your mind with peace.
All anxieties must go
That's not set in stone.

Worries become unsolved problems.
That will torment us
And will cause sickness.

Annoyed, mentally exhausted.
Unstable to handle problems.
No one can be worry-free.

Worries will not go away.
Most worries are fixed to life.
Stay focused on the right choices.

Control worries.
Circumstances will continue to arise
To become unsolved problems.

Our future, not told to us.
Prepare for tomorrow
And our worries.

Will still be with us
To the end.

Without Light

11-21-2012

Midnight light glows
Till morning draws
The night darkness.

Without light, we cannot see.
We need light to see.
Where our feet may go.

Our minds illuminated
By God's words of light
With understanding.

We see clearly now.
We need the words of light.
The word beams of light.

From the darkness
Of the night with no light.
Spiritually darkened by the night lights.

We live in the shadows of darkness.
To live without light.
Would be to live in darkness.

We cannot see in darkness.
Without the light of the truth.
That we seek.

The truth.
The words of God.
We walk in the light.

You Say

8-30-2012

What we say.
We utter words
That destroy one another.

Words get to feelings
And cut like a knife.
You bleed from the inside.

Speaking words with
No feeling of love.
You say that you love me.

Your words do not speak love.
They only spread hate.
Confused between love and hate.

What can we do?
With these words.
Words cannot be taken back.

What's already been said.
Try to do something.
To make up for what's been said.

There's nothing left to say.
You have already said enough.

www.ingramcontent.com/pod-product-compliance
Lightning Source LLC
Chambersburg PA
CBHW021644120626